Copyright © 2020 by Maure

All rights reserved. No part of this publication may be reproduced, distributed, or transmitted in any form or by any means, including photocopying, recording, or other electronic or mechanical methods, without the prior written permission of the publisher, except in the case of brief quotations embodied in critical reviews and certain other noncommercial uses permitted by copyright law.

The purpose of this book is to assist readers become well informed healthcare consumers. It is provided as overall health care advice.

It is always suggested that you seek medical advice from your personal physician before starting any fresh workout program.

This book is not designed to be a replacement for a certified physician's medical recommendation. In all issues pertaining to his / her health, the reader should check with their doctor. **Note:** This is a book and not a product. Be guided!

Table of Contents

The Black Seed Oil 4
- Black Seed Oil Safety 8
- Uses of Black Seed Oil 9
- Health Benefits of Black Seed Oil 14
- Benefits of Black Seed Oil to the Skin 17
- Benefits of Black Seed Oil for Eczema 18
- Benefits of Black seed oil for Acne 20
- Benefits of Black Seed Oil for Allergies 23
- Benefits of Black Seed Oil for Cancer 24
- Benefits of Black Seed Oil for Candida 25
- Benefits of Black Seed Oil for Constipation 25
- Benefits of Black Seed Oil for Diabetes 25
- Benefits of Black Seed Oil for Epilepsy 26
- Benefits of Black Seed Oil for Estrogen 27
- Benefits of Black Seed Oil for Fibromyalgia 27
- Benefits of Black Seed Oil for Hair growth 28
- Benefits of Black Seed Oil for High blood pressure 29
- Benefits of Black Seed Oil for Inflammation 30
- Benefits of Black Seed Oil for Lyme disease 31
- Benefits of Black Seed Oil for Menopause 34
- Benefits of Black Seed Oil for Nausea 34
- Benefits of Black Seed Oil for Pets 35
- Benefits of Black Seed Oil for Pregnancy 36

Benefits of Black Seed Oil for Weight loss 38
  Benefits of Black Seed Oil with Raw Honey 38
Potential Side effects of Black seed oil 40
Special Precautions & Warnings: 41
Black Seed Oil Dosing Considerations 42
How to Buy Black Seed Oil 48

The Black Seed Oil

Plants have long been used in the history of mankind as the basis of traditional remedies, and even serve as sources of modern medicines. For their primary health care needs, more than three-fourths of populations in resource-limited countries rely on medicinal plants as more than 60% of societies are unable to access and/or afford allopathic medicines. In line with the latest developments in the field of optimal nutrition, interest in the use of plants as a source of food and medicine is now resurgent. Recently, the usage of phytomedicine has been amplified dramatically for numerous ailments because of not only their easy accessibility and low cost but also the belief that natural remedies have fewer harmful effects as compared to synthetic medicines.

This is also encouraged to create new medicines from natural sources as it is estimated that only 15 percent of the 300,000 herbal species that exist globally have been investigated for their pharmacological potential. Nigella sativa L, with many medicinal plants

(Ranunculaceae) has been considered one of the most treasured nutrient-rich herbs in the world's history and numerous scientific studies are underway to verify the historically claimed uses of this species 'small seed

Black seed oil is extracted from the seeds of Nigella sativa, a plant native to southwest Asia. The black seeds are slightly bitter and sometimes used as a flavoring or spice in Middle Eastern and Indian cuisine. The amber-hued oil is also used in cooking and is said to offer a range of health benefits. One of the key components of black seed oil is thymoquinone, a compound with antioxidant properties.

The seeds have been used for healing and protection for thousands of years. More recently black seed oil has been shown to have antioxidant properties which could reduce inflammation inside the body if consumed.

Black seed oil has a long history of use dating back over 2000 years. According to some sources it was discovered in the tomb of King Tutankhamen, an ancient Egyptian pharaoh. The oil is used by some for the treatment of conditions including asthma, diabetes, hypertension, weight loss, and other conditions. There is scientific evidence to support some, but not all, uses for black seed oil.

While using black seeds in small amounts in cooking can be a tasty way of incorporating the seeds in your diet, large-scale clinical trials are needed before the oil can be recommended as a treatment for any condition.

It is very crucial for you to seek the Advice or help of an expert before ingesting black seed oil or using it topically

If you're still thinking of using black seed oil for health purposes, be sure to speak with your healthcare provider first to weigh the pros and cons and discuss whether it's right for you.

Black seed oil is known by several names including:

- Black cumin seed oil
- Kalonji oil

- Nigella sativa oil
- Ajenuz, Aranuel
- Baraka
- Black Caraway
- Charnuska
- Cheveux de Vénus
- Cominho Negro
- Comino Negro,
- Cumin Noir
- Cyah Dane
- Fennel Flower
- Fitch
- Graine de Nigelle
- Graine Noire
- Habatul Sauda,
- Habbatul Baraka
- Kalajaji
- Kalajira
- Kalonji,
- Ketsah,
- La Grainer Noire,
- Love in a Mist
- Mugrela

- Nielle
- Nutmeg Flower
- Roman-Coriander

Black Seed Oil Safety

It's possible that black seed oil can increase the effects of medicines that the body processes through the cytochrome P450 pathway. Enzymes in this pathway metabolize 90 percent of common medications. Examples of common medications can include beta-blockers such as metoprolol (Lopressor) and the blood thinner warfarin (Coumadin).

If you take any prescription medications regularly, talk to your doctor before starting to take black seed oil. You shouldn't stop taking any of your regular medications without talking to your doctor first.

Black seed oil can be helpful to liver function, but taking too much black seed oil can also be harmful to your liver and kidneys. If you have problems with either of these organs, talk to your doctor to determine a safe dose (if any). Also, topical black seed oil can cause allergic reactions. Do a patch test before applying it to a large area on your skin.

Uses of Black Seed Oil

Used in cosmetic and topical applications, Black Cumin Seed Oil can be applied directly to the preferred areas of skin to hydrate, to soothe acne, burns, and other unwanted blemishes, and to reduce the appearance of the signs of aging, such as fine lines. Alternatively, 2 drops of Black Cumin Seed Carrier Oil can be added to a regular, pre-made face cream of personal preference. Applying a moisturizer infused with this oil is also known to address fungus and skin infections.

For a moisturizer that offers the added benefits of several other nutrient-rich oils, combine the following ingredients in a dark, clean 105 ml (3.5 oz.) dropper bottle:

1. Jojoba Carrier Oil 30 ml (1 oz.)
2. Sweet Almond Carrier Oil 30 ml (1 oz.)
3. Borage Carrier Oil 20 ml (0.7 oz.)
4. Rosehip Carrier Oil 15 ml (0.5 oz.)

5. Black Cumin Seed Carrier Oil 9 ml (0.3 oz.)
6. Vitamin E Liquid. 6 ml (0.02 oz.)

Cap the bottle and shake it gently to ensure that all the oils have mixed together thoroughly. Before applying this blend, cleanse the face and pat it dry, leaving it slightly damp to the touch. Next, warm up 6-8 drops of this elixir by rubbing this amount between the palms, and then gently massage it into the face and neck using light strokes in an upward motion. Avoid applying the blend around the eye area. Due to the absence of preservatives in this formulation, it should be used within 6 months of the day it is made.

For a nourishing, protective Black Cumin Seed Oil face mask that functions as an exfoliating scrub to buff away dead skin, begin by cleansing the face with a gentle face wash and ensure that all traces of makeup have been removed. Next, in a small dish or bowl mix,

- 1 Tbsp. Black Cumin Seed Carrier Oil
- 3 Tbsp. Raw Organic Honey
- 3 Tbsp. Finely-ground Apricot Shell exfoliator.

Use the fingertips to apply the mask, gently smoothing 1 Tbsp. of the blend (this recipe yields approximately 7 Tbsp.) into the face and neck in a circular motion. After the mask has soaked into the skin for 10 minutes, massage it deeper into the skin while rinsing it off with warm water. Pat the skin dry, then moisturize with 1-2 drops of Black Cumin Seed Carrier Oil. This mask is known to purify the skin, reduce the appearance of blemishes, and smooth the look of wrinkles to promote an even complexion with a healthy glow.

For a stimulating and conditioning hair mask that is reputed to nourish hair and enhance its growth while soothing the scalp, first pour 2 Tbsp. of Black Cumin Seed Carrier Oil onto the palms of the hands and rub them together to warm the oil. Next, massage the entire scalp with this amount of oil, focusing particularly on the areas that are experiencing the most hair loss. Once the oil has been massaged into the entire scalp, smooth the oil down over the strands all the way to the tips. Leave the hair mask in for 30-60 minutes, after which time it can be rinsed out with a regular shampoo. This mask is known to strengthen and support scalp health, reduce hair loss, eliminate dandruff, prevent dryness, balance the scalp's oil production, reduce frizz, protect the strands against damage, and prevent hair from losing its pigmentation, thereby slowing the graying process. This regimen can be repeated 2-3 times a week.

Used in medicinal applications, Black Cumin Seed Oil is reputed to be beneficial for a wide range of ailments and conditions, but it is best known for its ability to ease joint pain, muscle aches, bruises, and symptoms of rheumatism. For a simple yet effectively restorative massage that works to repair skin damage and reduce skin discoloration caused by bruises, gently massage 60 ml (2 oz.) of Black Cumin Seed Carrier Oil into affected areas, focusing particularly on bruising and uneven skin tone. This can be repeated 2-3 times a day until the soreness and inflammation have been eliminated and the color returns to normal. This is also reputed to be beneficial for eczema and acne. Furthermore, it energizes tired muscles, strengthens immunity, reduces stiffness, eases digestive complaints, promotes the expulsion of bodily toxins, and regulates menstruation as well as related complaints.

For a diffuser recipe that is known to provide relief from nasal congestion, sore throat, headache, and other cold symptoms, diffuse 2 drops of Black Cumin Seed Carrier Oil. Its comforting scent is known to ease nervous tension and lethargy. To enhance the effects of this steam inhalation regimen, 2 drops of the oil can also be massaged onto the affected areas, such as the neck and chest, to relieve aches, clear the respiratory tract, and soothe irritation.

Health Benefits of Black Seed Oil

Although research on the health effects of black seed oil is fairly limited, there's some evidence that it may offer certain benefits. Here's a look at several key findings from available studies

Rheumatoid Arthritis

Black seed oil may aid in the treatment of rheumatoid arthritis, according to a small study published in Immunological Investigations in 2016, 43 women with mild-to-moderate rheumatoid arthritis took black seed oil capsules or a placebo every day for one month.

Results showed that treatment with black seed oil led to a reduction in arthritis symptoms (as assessed by the DAS-28 rating scale), blood levels of inflammatory markers, and the number of swollen joints.

Nasal Inflammation

Black seed oil shows promise in the treatment of allergies. In a 2011 study published in the American

Journal of Otolaryngology, for instance, black seed oil was found to reduce the presence of nasal congestion and itching, runny nose, and sneezing after two weeks.

Another report published in 2018 analyzed data to determine if black seed oil could help in the treatment of sinusitis. There was a conclusion that the oil has therapeutic potential in the treatment of the condition due to its anti-inflammatory, antioxidant, antihistaminic, immune-modulator, antimicrobial, and analgesic effects.

Diabetes

Black seed oil may be of some benefit to people with diabetes, Researchers analyzed previously published studies on the use of Nigella sativa for diabetes and concluded that it could improve blood sugar and cholesterol levels in diabetes models but noted that clinical trials are necessary to clarify the effects.

Asthma

Black seed oil may offer benefits to people with asthma. For example, a study published in Phytotherapy Research in 2017 found that people with asthma who took black seed oil capsules had a significant improvement in asthma control compared with those who took a placebo.

Obesity

Black seed oil may reduce risk factors in women who are obese.

According to a study, women consumed Nigella sativa oil or a placebo while following a low-calorie diet for eight weeks. At the study's end, weight, waist circumference, and triglyceride levels had decreased by more in the group that took the Nigella sativa oil.

Another eight-week study combined aerobic exercise with black seed oil in a trial with overweight sedentary women. Researchers found that the exercise protocol paired with supplementation provided benefits including lower cholesterol levels

Other Uses

Black seed oil is also used as a remedy for conditions such as allergies, diabetes, headaches, high blood pressure, and digestive disorders.

In addition, black seed oil is said to boost the immune system, reduce inflammation, and fight infections. The oil is used topically for skin and hair concerns, such as acne, dry hair, psoriasis, hair growth, and dry skin.

Benefits of Black Seed Oil to the Skin

Black cumin has many benefits when you apply the oil topically. The one that really sticks out as being different from many other plant ingredients is the oil's powerful ability to restore the look and vibrancy of your skin.

Nourishes

Black cumin provides vitamins A, B, and C, along with minerals like calcium, potassium, magnesium, and zinc, giving skin what it needs to be healthy.

Reduces oily skin and clogged pores

This oil has a reputation as helping to help with oily skin. If you're struggling with too much oil and clogged pores, you need to try this oil.

Moisturizes

Like many natural oils, black cumin seed oil is rich in essential fatty acids that provide deep, lasting moisturization for skin. These fatty acids also help reduce the appearance of fine lines and wrinkles.

Reduces the appearance of dark spots

Regular application of this oil will help to reduce the appearance of dark spots. Vitamin A and amino acids together with fatty acids help to encourage a youthful look.

Benefits of Black Seed Oil for Eczema

Eczema is an unpleasant skin condition that can cause a lot of discomfort in sufferers. It typically manifests as dry, rough patches of skin which can be very itchy and sometimes painful. In more severe cases these patches can become scaly or hard and start to ooze. There are a number of topical options for treating eczema and the most common treatment is steroid creams. However, these products are often made from synthetic materials and pose some potential risks to the user. For those looking to improve their eczema with a natural and highly effective product, black seed oil is the ideal choice.

How Black Seed Oil Helps Eczema

Black seed oil helps to improve eczema in a number of ways. When used externally and applied directly to affected skin, the oil works to soothe patches right away. The oil is naturally anti-inflammatory which helps to reduce swelling and redness and to minimize discomfort caused by inflammation. It also contains fatty acids, including omega-3, which helps to moisturize the skin. This makes the oil very soothing and not only reduces the pain and itch associated with dryness but also works to soften skin that has become thick or hardened. Black seed oil also contains zinc, potassium, and B vitamins which all contribute to hydration and healing of skin.

Taking black seed oil internally can be helpful in the battle against eczema as well. Eczema is generally considered to be the result of a faulty immune system in which certain immune proteins mistakenly target the body's own tissues. Black seed oil is great for supporting the immune system and helps to balance it without increasing reactions against healthy tissue. Some eczema is suspected to be relates to allergies and can still be soothed using black seed oil as it is a natural anti-histamine that reduces the allergic reactions that cause dry, itchy skin patches.

Benefits of Black seed oil for Acne

Acne isn't just a skin-deep problem. It's been documented that people with acne struggle more with depression than people without it. Acne strips people of their confidence and makes them feel like no one can see the real them. Simply put, having acne, whether it's mild, severe or somewhere in between, is no walk in the park.

There are four main factors behind acne:

- Oil (or sebum)

- Dead skin cells
- Bacteria
- Clogged pores

Acne is caused by an abundance of oil and dead skin cells clumping together in your pores. Pores are also hair follicles, so a person with acne basically has oil and skin cells stuck in their hair follicles. That clogged pore/hair follicle is the ideal environment for bacteria to thrive in.

Black cumin seeds contain over 100 chemical compounds, many of which have a direct, positive effect on the skin. For example, thymoquinone (TQ) is an active ingredient in black cumin seeds. TQ is anti-inflammatory. What this means is that inflamed acne bumps, whether they are painful or not, can be treated by rubbing black cumin seed oil on them.

Black cumin is high in zinc, which fights infections and clears acne.

Black cumin is also a potent antibacterial agent. A research paper published in 2008 showed that black cumin seed oil was nearly as effective at fighting bacteria as many prescription antibiotics.

In the experiment, varying strengths of black cumin oil were tested against different types of bacteria. For the control, researchers also tested the effectiveness of a number of popular antibiotics to see how well they worked against the same bacteria.

What they found was nothing short of incredible. Out of 144 strains of bacteria, the researchers found that 97 of them were stopped in their tracks by black cumin seed oil. Black cumin was found to be even more effective than the antibiotics for treating certain types of bacteria.

This is the thing that acne sufferers need to know; some of the antibiotics tested, like erythromycin, are regularly used to treat acne.

While more study is needed, this research is still incredibly helpful in understanding why black cumin seed oil can be effective in fighting bacteria that is normally resistant to medication and treatment. This could be particularly helpful for treating acne that resists antibiotics.

Benefits of Black Seed Oil for Allergies

When your immune system reacts to something that is normally harmless, you have an allergy. From a runny nose and watering eyes all the way through to anaphylactic shock and death is what can result from allergies. Wouldn't it be great if we had at our disposal a cheap and effective method to stop the immune system from overreacting?

We have known about black seed's ability as an anti-histamine from as far back as 1970. A significant anti-histamine effect was found. "An inhaled thymoquinone aerosol dose-dependently protected guinea pigs against histamine-stimulated bronchospasm in the range of 2.5–10 mg/kg"

There is more research on black seed being an anti-histamine but it's mainly been performed in relation to asthma. I did, however, find a bunch of patents for allergy products that include black seed as a constituent for alleviating symptoms.

Benefits of Black Seed Oil for Cancer

The antitumor activity of thymoquinone and thymohydroquinone in mice and discovered that the two phytochemicals in black seed oil can result in 52% decrease in tumor cells!

Being rich in both chemicals, black seed is unique in that it can help prevent and treat cancer through a variety of mechanisms:

- Anti-proliferation
- Apoptosis induction
- Cell cycle arrest
- Reactive oxygen species generation
- Anti-metastasis
- Anti-angiogenesis

The anti-tumor effects of thymoquinone have also been investigated in tumor xenograft mice models for colon, prostate, pancreatic and lung cancer. The combination of thymoquinone and conventional chemotherapeutic drugs could produce greater therapeutic effect as well as reduce the toxicity of the latter.

Benefits of Black Seed Oil for Candida

Black seed oil helps fight Candida overgrowth, thrush and fungal infections in the digestive tract and on the skin. In thrush it can be used both internally and externally.

Benefits of Black Seed Oil for Constipation

Black cumin seeds and oil are carminative, which means they can support digestion and decrease digestive problems including gas, bloating, and stomach pain.

Benefits of Black Seed Oil for Diabetes

Nigella sativa oil causes gradual partial regeneration of pancreatic beta-cells, increases the lowered serum insulin concentrations and decreases the elevated serum glucose. It means that Black seed is one of the few remedies that could help prevent and treat not type 2 but also type 1 diabetes in which own immune system destroys insulin producing pancreatic beta cells.

In addition, Nigella sativa improves glucose tolerance as efficiently as metformin; yet it has not shown significant adverse effects and has very low toxicity.

Black Seed Oil supplementation improves insulin sensitivity and helps maintain normal blood sugar level. In addition, Nigella sativa reduced levels of glycosylated hemoglobin (HbA1c). Our systematic review revealed that N. sativa supplementation might be effective in glycemic control in humans."

Benefits of Black Seed Oil for Epilepsy

Nigella sativa was able to prevent seizures and convulsions (in several animal studies) and had anti-epileptic activity in children through its neuroprotective, anti-inflammatory, calming & stress-relieving effect.

Benefits of Black Seed Oil for Estrogen

Nigella sativa possesses estrogenic function in the ovariectomized rat model which can be helpful in managing menopausal symptoms as an alternative for Hormone Replacement Therapy.

Nigella sativa exert estrogenic effect were exhibited through luteotropic assay and vaginal cell cornification as well as blood estrogen level. Furthermore, low dose Nigella sativa, methanol extract and linoleic acid had prominent estrogenic like effects which were significantly different from those of control group in different experiments.

Benefits of Black Seed Oil for Fibromyalgia

Fibromyalgia is a chronic pain disorder that causes pain and tenderness all-over the body. Injury, stress, and a family history of the condition can trigger the pain.

One of the most powerful (and yet too often overlooked) options is nigella sativa, also known as black cumin. This medicinal herb contains a powerful healing oil capable of quelling systemic inflammation and soothing chronic pain. Adding nigella sativa to one's dietary repertoire is easy, safe, and highly effective: and there are at least 900 peer-reviewed scientific articles that have been published over the years to prove it

Nigella sativa can mean the difference between endless suffering (when you don't take it) and sustained relief (when you do). The many natural phytochemicals contained in nigella sativa have been scientifically shown to help keep inflammation levels in check; promote healthy weight; ward off harmful pathogens; support brain health; fight cancer cells; balance blood sugar; improve hair and skin health; and boost quality of life.

Benefits of Black Seed Oil for Hair growth

Probably one of the most unique black seed oil benefits is its uncanny ability to help restore hair loss. No one quite understands why it happens, but it's not too hard to guess that it has something to do with its powerful antioxidant and antimicrobial properties. By strengthening hair follicles, there is very good reason to see how black seed oil can help promote strengthened hair roots.

Benefits of Black Seed Oil for High blood pressure

Diet is a major risk factor, with eating lots of salty foods shown to increase risk. However, consuming black seed oil may help lower elevated blood pressure. It has been shown that taking black cumin seed extract for two months could reduce blood pressure readings in people whose blood pressure was slightly elevated.

In addition to lowering high blood pressure, it can reduce risk of a heart attack. It contains high levels of fatty acids such as linoleic acids and oleic acid which work to reduce high cholesterol. Additionally, it could help relieve symptoms of an upset tummy. Though, black seed oil needn't always be eaten for its multiple benefits.

Benefits of Black Seed Oil for Inflammation

Inflammation can do a lot of damage, but not all inflammation is harmful, some is part of a healthy defense against malignant cells, infection and trauma, at least to a degree. When inflammation becomes systemic and chronic that is when true damage occurs as it can harms cells and lead to mutations; nearly a quarter of all cancers can be attributed to this inflammatory process. Maintaining balance between healthy and destructive inflammation can be important to avoiding disease, but with age the natural balance can be disrupted. Black cumin seed oil may be of benefit in this regard as the seeds of black cumin have a powerful antioxidant phytochemical in it called thymoquinone, and an antimicrobial and antiseptic called thymol.

Black cumin seed oil has been shown to increase activity of macrophages that surround and destroy abnormal cells in the body, and help to stimulate helper T-cells that facilitate healing. One study showed those who took black cumin seed oil had a

30% increase in natural killer cell functions and 55% increase in helper T-cell activity.

Benefits of Black Seed Oil for Lyme disease

Lyme disease is a debilitating disease transmitted by spirochete bacteria. It is often caused by lxodes ticks (deer ticks), and found in wooded and grassy areas. Most people think that this disease is common only in U.S. East Coast area. But, in reality, it is quite common throughout the United Stated and in many other countries.

Unfortunately, there is currently no credible vaccine to treat this disease. Therefore, its cases have been trending upward. This disease is indeed spreading in new areas and affecting people on a grand scale. Nigella Sativa is an annual flowering plant in the family Ranunculaceae. Its flowers contain pod that carry many seeds, known as 'black seeds' and 'black cumin'. They have a strong aroma and taste with notes of onion and black pepper.

The healing power of Nigella Sativa is quite unbelievable. Especially, when it comes to treating

Lyme disease, its potent compounds, like thymoquinone, work with efficacy. Thymoquinone is one of those special compounds that have been widely studied by the scientists. It is a potent antioxidant agent that treats allergy, inflammation, and immune response. For that reason, it has the ability to cure Lyme within a few days!

Particularly, in Nigella Sativa oil (black seed oil) form, it is famous for killing Lyme bacteria. Apart from this, thymoquinone also inhibits NF-kappaB. This group of protein is associated with inflammation and autoimmune disorders. In a way, thymoquinone works on the roots of the Lyme and banishes it from your body forever. Many Lyme disease victims have used it for their quick recoveries. Unlike other herbal oils, it doesn't only treat Lyme, but also your entire body. If you are dealing with chronic, severe third-stage symptoms, you can count on this compound to treat Lyme.

Also, your immune system plays a significant role in treating Lyme disease. Several studies have detected antibodies, produce by immune system, which kill those bacteria that cause Lyme. In other words, if you have a strong and healthy immune system, it won't let this disease affect any organ or system inside the body.

Luckily, the positive effects of Nigella Sativa on the immune system are astounding. It is a natural immune enhancer that plays an important role in treating the deadliest diseases associated with immune system. When taken properly, your body turns into a fortress against Lyme disease.

It was confirm that it boosts the production of white blood cells. These cells assist your body in preventing Lyme. They in fact wipe out those harmful bacteria that antibiotic medications cannot. Therefore, herbalists often recommend Nigella Sativa oil for Lyme treatment. According to them, its internal and external application makes it more potent and effective than other natural herbs.

Benefits of Black Seed Oil for Menopause

Black seed oil is used in the treatment of postmenopausal symptoms and is plausible to be an alternative to hormone replacement therapy (HRT) for post menopause in human.

Benefits of Black Seed Oil for Nausea

Black seed oil for nausea and upset stomachs are another notorious use of black seeds.

The reason why it makes for such a powerful remedy for the occasional non-debilitating nausea or upset stomach is due to the fact that it stimulates your body's digestion and induces the expulsion of gas both two natural processes of a healthy person.

For nausea, a common recipe is mixing a teaspoon of black seed oil with a teaspoon of ginger juice (twice daily).

For chronic or debilitating nausea or upset stomach, seek medical attention immediately.

Benefits of Black Seed Oil for Pets

Black Seed Oil is a herbs for pet product known for its antibiotic, anti-oxidant, anti-inflammatory and anticancer properties. Many health experts claim that it is, indeed, a true panacea; able to help cure everything from allergies to hypertension. It is a safe, plant-based viable alternative to conventional supplements and can be beneficial for:

- Killing multi-drug resistant "superbugs" associated with viral and bacterial infection, including TB
- Eliminating fungus and mold
- Reducing inflammation and relieving associated pain due to arthritis or injury
- Providing antioxidant support to fight free radical damage that could lead to cancer
- Preserving antioxidant enzymes that protect the liver and aid cellular antioxidant defense systems

Ingredients: Black Seed Oil, Fermented Cod Liver Oil, Frankincense, Myrrh Oil

Suggested Use: two times daily for 10- 30 days then once a day for 6 days a week as needed

Benefits of Black Seed Oil for Pregnancy

For general fertility health, black seed oil can help support a healthy reproductive system and healthy levels of fertility.

Antioxidant components in medicinal herbs such as Nigella sativa (NS) have been studied to determine if they improve spermatogenesis and steroidogenesis.

A study published in the Journal of Herbal Medicine aimed to study the effects of Nigella sativa on male infertility.

The outcome of this study indicated that Nigella Sativa can possibly influence sperm parameters, semen, Leydig cells, reproductive organs and sexual hormones, although there was no conclusive evidence of full improvement.

The main potential mechanism of use is through the antioxidant properties of Nigella Sativa. Thymoquinone (TQ) and unsaturated fatty acids are the main antioxidant components of Nigella Sativa.

Although the findings of this review suggest that Nigella Sativa is a potential candidate for male infertility treatment, there is insufficient evidence to make recommendations for its use as an adjunct therapy in infertile men.

Infertility can have a variety of different causes and is best consulted with a doctor.

More clinical trials are recommended to demonstrate the efficacy of Nigella Sativa on male infertility.

With a healthy diet and workout, black seed oil may act as a natural aphrodisiac. With the help of blood circulation and oxygen to sex organs, your sex drive may improve.

Benefits of Black Seed Oil for Weight loss

Black seed oil weight loss claims actually do have some science behind them. The Journal of Diabetes and Metabolic Disorders published a study systemically reviewing the literature for plants that have anti-obesity properties and discovered that black seed oil was among the most effective natural remedies on the planet.

Benefits of Black Seed Oil with Raw Honey

First we should not forget that nothing works alone. If you live a life in hate and envy, eat junk food and don't exercise, but eat black seeds, don't expect to be cured anytime soon. The cure comes first from the inside of your spirit, then from your life-style. Make peace with yourself and the world, and then help your body with good natural medicine like the black seeds. In a good environment, the body has everything needed to heal itself.

We can find Nigella Sativa in two forms on the market: as raw seeds or as oil (encapsulated or bottled).

1 teaspoon of oil = 2.5 teaspoons of powdered seeds

It was part of the tradition to put some honey and ground whole black seeds in the palm of your right hand and lick it up with your tongue. In the days of Prophet Mohammad, he was taking them like that; there was no black seed oil back then.

The protocol:

Combine 1 teaspoon of oil with 1 teaspoon of raw honey (or freshly squeezed juice) and take them 3 times per day.

One with half an hour before breakfast, one in the afternoon and one just before bedtime.

You can replace the oil with the seeds, only that they need to be heated first (otherwise it will burn your stomach) and then ground. Put the seeds in a frying pan on a very low heat and stir them from time to time. When their flavor is gone take them off and ground them.

Potential Side effects of Black seed oil

When taken by mouth: When taken in small quantities, such as a flavoring for foods, black seed is likely safe for most people. Black seed oil and black seed powder are possibly safe when the larger amounts found in medicine are used for 3 months or less. There isn't enough reliable information to know if the amounts found in medicine are safe when used for more than 3 months. Black seed can cause allergic rashes in some people. It can also cause stomach upset, vomiting, or constipation. It might increase the risk of seizures in some people.

When applied to the skin: Black seed oil or gel is possibly safe when applied to the skin, short-term. It can cause allergic rashes in some people.

Special Precautions & Warnings:

Pregnancy and breast-feeding: Black seed seems to be safe in food amounts during pregnancy. But taking the larger amounts found in medicine is **likely unsafe**. Black seed can slow down or stop the uterus from contracting.

There isn't enough reliable information to know if black seed is safe to use when breast-feeding. Stay on the safe side and avoid use.

Children: Black seed oil is **possibly safe** for children when taken by mouth short-term and in recommended amounts.

Bleeding disorders: Black seed might slow blood clotting and increase the risk of bleeding. In theory, black seed might make bleeding disorders worse.

Diabetes: Black seed might lower blood sugar levels in some people. Watch for signs of low blood sugar (hypoglycemia) and monitor your blood sugar carefully if you have diabetes and use black seed.

Low blood pressure: Black seed might lower blood pressure. In theory, taking black seed might make blood pressure become too low in people with low blood pressure.

Surgery: Black seed might slow blood clotting, reduce blood sugar, and increase sleepiness in some people. In theory, black seed might increase the risk for bleeding and interfere with blood sugar control and anesthesia during and after surgical procedures. Stop using black seed at least two weeks before a scheduled surgery.

Black Seed Oil Dosing Considerations

The correct dosage of any supplement requires a comprehensive analysis of many factors including your age, sex, health conditions, DNA, and lifestyle.

- For opiate addiction, 500 mg of dried black seeds has been used three times daily for up to twelve days.

- For allergies, 40-80 mg/kg daily of black seed oil has been used three times daily for up to eight weeks.
- For anxiety, half a teaspoon of Nigella sativa oil has been taken with herbal tea based on traditional use.
- For arthritis, one teaspoon of Nigella sativa oil with one teaspoon of olive oil has been administered three times a day for arthritis, based on traditional use.
- For bruises, one teaspoon of Nigella sativa oil with one teaspoon of olive oil has been taken three times daily, based on traditional use.
- For cold symptoms, based on traditional use, 1 teaspoon of Nigella sativa oil has been ingested three times a daily.
- For diabetes, Nigella sativa oil 2.5mL twice daily for six weeks, in addition to existing metformin, has been used.
- For diarrhea, based on traditional use, 1 teaspoon of Nigella sativa oil with a cup of yogurt has been taken twice daily.

- For headache, based on traditional use, 1/2 tsp. of Nigella sativa oil has been drunk after a meal three times daily.
- For hyperlipidemia, Nigella sativa oil 2.5mL twice daily for six weeks, in addition to existing antilipemic agents, has been used.
- For hypertension, 100 and 200 mg of boiled extract has been taken twice daily for eight weeks. Based on traditional use, 1 tsp. of Nigella sativa oil has been drunk in any hot drink and taken with two cloves of garlic before breakfast.
- For influenza, based on traditional use, 1 tsp. of Nigella sativa oil has been taken three times daily.
- For muscle soreness, based on traditional use, 1 tsp. of Nigella sativa oil with 1 tsp. of olive oil has been taken three times daily.
- For respiratory disorders, Nigella sativa aqueous boiled extract (0.375mL/kg of a 50mg/mL solution) for two months has been used.

- For asthma, 15mL/kg of a 0.1% boiled extract has been taken daily for three months. For asthma, 50 or 100 mg/kg of boiled extract Nigella sativa has been also used. Based on traditional use, the back and chest have also been rubbed with Nigella sativa oil. Inhalation of vapor of boiling water with 1 tsp. of Nigella sativa oil with a towel over the head has been implemented.
- For rheumatic diseases, based on traditional use, 1 tsp. of Nigella sativa oil with 1 tsp. of olive oil has been ingested three times daily.
- For Sinusitis, based on traditional use, 1 tsp. of Nigella sativa oil has been taken daily in chronic sinusitis cases; in acute sinusitis cases, 1 tsp. of Nigella sativa oil has been taken three times daily.
- For stomach disorders, based on traditional use, mint tea with lemon has been ingested with 1 tsp. of Nigella sativa oil three times a day or until symptoms are relieved.
- For alopecia (hair loss), based on traditional use, first the scalp is stroked thoroughly with

lemon, left for 15 minutes, then washed and dried; then 1/2-1 tsp. of Nigella sativa oil is applied.

- As an antifungal (applied to the skin), based on traditional use, the affected area is wiped with cider vinegar; then Nigella sativa oil is applied and repeated if necessary.
- For atopic dermatitis, an ointment containing 15% black seed oil has been applied for four weeks without evidence of benefit. For colic, based on traditional use, Nigella sativa oil is warmed in the hand; then the whole abdomen is massaged.
- For cough, based on traditional use, the back and chest is rubbed with Nigella sativa oil. Inhalation of vapor of boiling water with 1 tsp. of Nigella sativa oil with a towel over the head has also been used.
- For earache, based on traditional use, 1/2 tsp. of Nigella sativa oil is mixed with 1/2 tsp. of olive oil; then it is warmed and dripped into the ear; then a hat or scarf is placed over the ear.

- For headache, based on traditional use, the forehead and sides of the head and part of the face near the ears are rubbed with Nigella sativa oil.
- For acne, based on traditional use, inhalation of vapor of hot water with 1/2 tsp. of Nigella sativa oil with a towel over the head has been used.
- For sinusitis, based on traditional use, inhalation of Nigella sativa oil through the nose via a vapor bath has been used.
- For the treatment of allergies in children, 40-80 mg/kg daily of black seed oil has been used three times daily for up to eight weeks.
- For the treatment of epilepsy in children, aqueous extract of Nigella sativa seed (40 mg/kg per hour) has been used as an adjunct therapy for four weeks.

How to Buy Black Seed Oil

Widely available for purchase online, black seed oil is sold in many natural-foods stores and in stores specializing in dietary supplements.

When choosing oils, many consumers prefer to buy a product that is cold-pressed and organic to make sure that the oil is in its most natural state. Read labels carefully to make sure that other ingredients haven't been added to the product you choose.

Also, it's important to keep in mind that dietary supplements are largely unregulated by the FDA. It is not legal to market a dietary supplement product as a treatment or cure for a specific disease or to alleviate the symptoms of a disease. But the FDA does not test products for safety or effectiveness.

You may choose to look for familiar brands or products that have been certified by Consumer Labs, The U.S. Pharmacopeia Convention, or NSF International. These organizations don't guarantee that a product is safe or effective, but they do provide a certain level of testing for quality.

Printed in Great Britain
by Amazon